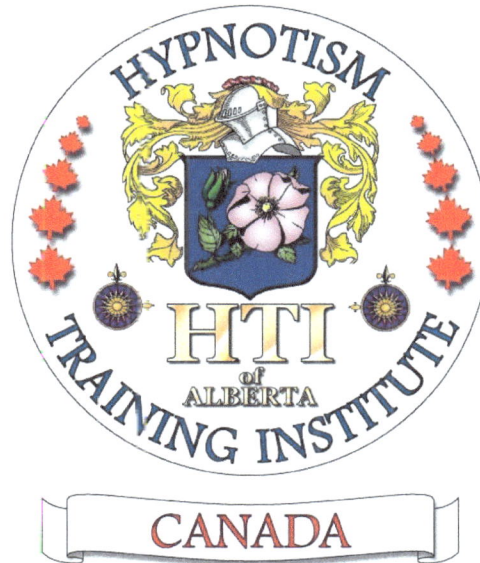

Hypnosis 202

Hypnotherapy:
Principle and Practice

By Anny J. Slegten

Hypnotherapy: Principle and Practice
Anny Slegten
Published by
Kimberlite Publishing House
www.kimberlitePublishingHouse.com

KIMBERLITE
PUBLISHING HOUSE

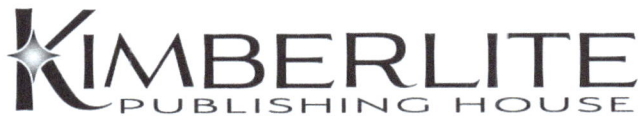

ISBN: 978-1-7752489-6-5

School Coat of Arms designed by Boomer Stralak
Book layout by Colin Christopher *www.colinchristopher.com*
Book cover and Kimberlite Logo designed by Marietta Miller
www.execugraphx.com

The Kimberlite-Diamond Connection

Kimberlite is a rock type that was first categorized over a 100 years ago based on descriptions of the diamond-bearing pipes of Kimberley, South Africa.

Kimberlites are the mechanism by which diamonds are brought to the surface.

Kimberlitic rocks are the most important primary source of diamonds and the main rock type in which significant diamond deposits have been found so far.

Anny is familiar with many rocks and minerals as her husband was raised around quarries, and later worked in several mines in Canada.

Therefore, it was natural for Anny to choose kimberlite as an analogy to the soul residing within our body – as a diamond within the kimberlite.

A Picture Is Worth A Thousand Words

The picture of my recliner on the book cover is a dedication to all my clients - young and old - who sat in this well used healing space.

One afternoon, a man, in his mid-twenties had a hypnotherapy session regarding his relationship with his father. At the end of his highly emotional and delightful hypnotherapy session he got up and looked at me.

Pointing at my recliner he declared "this is a magic chair!"

And since then, the picture of my recliner became my trademark.

With fond memories, I had to put my recliner in retirement, worn out after thirty-one year of constant use. When put in the reclining position I had to hold onto the chair to prevent it to flipping back on the floor.

The replacement arrived, and with great relief, I observed the magic side of the hypnotherapy sessions have been imparted to this comfortable new recliner.

With the aid of the magic recliner, private and surrogate sessions allow me to be current in my teaching and writings.

My wish is for you to have the privilege to facilitate the transformation of a soul. By taking these hypnosis and hypnotherapy courses, I hope you share in "The magic chair"

Anny

Welcome to

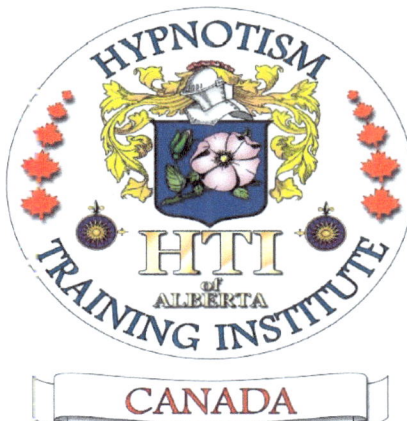

HYP 202 – Hypnotherapy: Principle and Practice

This book belongs to:

Name _____

Mailing Address _____

_____

City or Town _____

Province/State _____ Postal Code/Zip _____

Country _____

Telephone   Home (___) _____   Work (___) _____

Instructor's Name: ***Anny Slegten***

Today's Date: _____

Table Of Contents

A Note From Anny

The design and development of the Course Material required the investment of substantial effort, time and money and is only intended for the participants of HYP 202, Hypnotherapy: Principle & Practice.

Understand that the experiences derived from attending this course is a private and personal experience for each participant. As such please do respect the confidentiality of all participants and their remarks and actions and keep all such information private and confidential.

As a result, I am counting on you do your part at keeping this course environment safe and secure for all participants.

Enjoy!

Outline For HYP 202 Practical Exam

Purpose:

Appropriately formulate and give a suggestion requested by client.
It is important to have the client's assistance at writing this script.

First ask the client if at the end of the recording they want to fall asleep or want to come back to 'now'.

1-TOGETHER WITH YOUR CLIENT, FORMULATE A SUGGESTION.
Write it down.

2-LEAD THE CLIENT INTO A TRANCE.
Remember the client will be alone when listening to this recording.
Use an appropriated spoken induction.

3-SAY THE PRAYERS.

4-GIVE THE SUGGESTION <u>EXACTLY</u> AS FORMULATED.

5-DEEPEN THE TRANCE.
Use an appropriated induction since the client will be alone.

6-GIVE THE SUGGESTION AGAIN, <u>EXACTLY</u> AS FORMULATED.
By now, you may randomly choose and mix and match the written suggestion.

7-WRAP IT UP.
Choose from Anny's vernacular.

STOP THE RECORDING IF THEY WANT TO FALL ASLEEP LISTENING TO THE RECORDING.

8-BRING THE CLIENT BACK TO NOW (COMING OUT OF HYPNOSIS).

And now, I am going to count from 1 to 5 etc.

9-POST-HYPNOTIC INTERVIEW:
What surprised you?
What did you learn?

Transcript – How To Visualize

Gil: Hello this is Gil Boyne and welcome again to the Hypnotherapy Video Clinic. We are in Edmonds, Washington at the Hypnotism Training Institute of Washington with Director Charles Tebbits and we are going to do some work with some students today. Let us meet one now.

"Conrad, how are you? How can I help you today Conrad?"

Conrad: Umm, I would like to be able to visualize. I have heard that other people can do it and I have been working on it for a couple of years. I would say three years.

I have tried all the techniques people gave me and I do at times get pictures that I do not have control over those pictures. I would like to be able to do that, just to be able to do it. I think that I could probably function better with pictures.

Gil: It sounds almost like, I hear you saying that, so long as I cannot visualize, I have a reason not to realize the goals I set for myself. Or, once I learn to visualize, which I have not, then I will really be able to reach my goals.

Conrad: Yeah, yeah, okay.

Gil: Ha, ha, I have determined the other side of the coin too quickly. So now flop it over and say therefore since I cannot visualize, I cannot really blame myself or be blamed if I do not realize my goals as quickly as I would like to.

Your Notes

Anny's Teaching

Conrad: I never thought of it that way.

Gil: You will think of it that way now.

Conrad: Yeah, Yeah, that makes sense. A different dimension. I was looking at it clearly as a sensory thing. Not having anything to do with my progress in life.

Gil: First of all, it is a misnomer, there is a lot of things in this life that kind of become myths and yet myths are what we come to believe in. There are myths propagated by the government for example. Capitalistic democratic society....................

So, there are many myths that are propagated and yet we accept as facts. Let us come down more specifically to you. The myths that there is such a thing as a photographic memory and they will quote people, this person, there is a very famous story about a black male that was a railroad porter in the south. And visitors to town would be taken down to the railroad platform at a special time of day when these freight trains would come through.

This man who was illiterate would stand and watch the freight train had a twelve-digit number on the side, an identification number and it did go by with forty or fifty cars and he could recite every one of the twelve-digit numbers without a miss. He was actually kind of mentally retarded.

And people point to that and say see it is possible to have a photographic memory. That is not really the way it works. Those are anomalies. Those are things that are not representative of what is possible but just kind of phenomena, is a better way of saying it. And the saying, many people believe that they should be able to see when they close their eyes, whatever picture they direct.

Your Notes

Just as if they were watching it on a ten-foot television screen or motion picture screen. Something you would expect to see in three D. And that is not really true. Some people report that they do visualize in that way.

What I am going do in this demonstration is that I am going show you that you have perfect visualization capabilities. But in so doing, I want you to recognize that you are going to lose that alibi that you cannot fully realize your goals because you cannot not visualize.

Conrad: I will trade.

Gil: Ha, ha, it is a hell of a trade to make, is it not.

Induction by Gil Boyne:

Alright. Fix your gaze right here. Do not take your eyes from mine and just follow my instructions. Take a deep breath and fill up your lungs, exhale slowly. Eyelids heavy, droopy drowsy, sleepy. And now a second even deeper breath. Let it out slowly. Relax. Now a third deep breath. I will count from five down to one as I do your eyelids grow heavy, droopy, drowsy, sleepy. And by the time I reach the count of one they close right down you fall deeply into a slumber. Five, eyelids heavy, droopy, drowsy, and sleepy. Four the next time they blink that is hypnosis coming on you then. Three your heavy lids right closed. Two they begin closing, closing, closing, close them closing. One sleep and relax. Let every muscle and every nerve now begin to grow loose and limp and lazy. You are relaxing more with each sound that you hear. With each easy breath that you take. You are going deeper and deeper in drowsy relaxation. That is fine.

At some time in your life, you have seen a child's alphabet book. Perhaps when you were a child and perhaps again as an adult when you purchased such a book for a child or read such a book to a child. This alphabet book has on each page a letter of the alphabet and then an object is pictured. That object begins with the same letter that is printed up in the corner of the page. So, let us look at our alphabet book now and open it to the first page. The first letter is A. Tell me what object is pictured on that page.

Conrad: An apple.

Gil: An apple. What color is the apple?

Conrad: Red.

Gil: Red. What variety is the apple.

Conrad: MacIntosh.

Gil: How can you tell that?

Conrad: I do not know; I just know it.

Gil: You know it by the way it looks. Is not that it? What else is on the page other than an apple.

Conrad: A big letter A on the left-hand side of the page.

Gil: Is there anything else? Look and see if there is anything else. Is there something attached to the apple.?

Conrad: Oh, there is a stem and a little leaf.

Gil: A stem and a leaf. Alright. That is fine. Now I am going turn the page over. The letter is B what is the object?

Conrad: A bear.

Gil: Say it again (A bear). A bear. Alright. What color is the bear?

Conrad: It is brown.

Gil: It is a brown bear. Is it a great big fierce looking bear? Or a little bear cub? What kind of a bear is it?

Conrad: A teddy bear.

Gil: It is a teddy bear. It is a stuffed teddy bear. Let us go to the next page. The letter is C, what is the object in this picture?

Conrad: Cup

Gil: Alright what color is the cup?

Conrad: It is white.

Gil: A white cup. Is there anything else on the page or any decoration on the cup?

Conrad: A saucer.

Gil: Cup and a saucer. Now we will turn the page and we will come to the next letter which is D. What is the object on the page?

Conrad: It is a dog.

Gil: A dog. Is it a great big old mangy hound? Or some other kind of a dog?

Conrad: It is some kind of a terrier.

Gil: Alright, a small terrier, is that it?

Conrad: Yeah, bouncing around.

Gil: Is it an old dog or a young dog?

Conrad: Puppy.

Gil: It is a little puppy. Is there anything else on that page with the dog?

Conrad: The letter D.

Gil: The letter D. Is there anything else attached to the dog, connected to the dog?

Conrad: No.

Gil: Alright, fine. Were you able to see those clearly as pictures?

Conrad: No.

Gil: No, and yet you saw them some way, some how in your mind, didn't you? Yeah. So, you now begin to understand first that visualization is not necessarily occur on a screen or as if you are watching a screen. It is simply a knowing. Hum?

Conrad: Yes.

Gil: Alright, now here is what I want you to do. We are going to do this very simply just like a painter paints a canvas and puts in one element at a time.

You see. I want you now to just see one object and that is a bench. A park bench. Alright. Just become **aware** of a park bench. Sharp clear, defined... And when you are **aware** of the bench I want you to nod your head.

Alright? Now we are going to put that bench under a very large tree in the park and push it back up against the trunk of the tree. So now we will have the bench on the grass and the tree above and behind the bench. As soon as you are **aware** of the tree, nod your head.

Your Notes

Anny's Teaching

Alright. Now we are going to have a person on the bench, preferably you sitting there on the bench under the tree. As soon as you are **aware** of someone seated on the bench nod your head.

Now as you look out, on this bench, on the grass, under the tree, in the park a short distance away there is a kind of a gravel path that runs through the park. When you become **aware** of the gravel path nod your head.

Off to your right, as the path bends and goes around behind some shrubbery, as you look in that direction, coming right around that bend, here is a little boy coming along and in his right hand he is holding a balloon. The balloon he just bought, or his mother just bought for him from the vendors filled with helium and it is bobbing along as he walks and now he is coming down towards you and this boy has a head of beautiful red hair. And his face is covered with freckles. When you become **aware** of the boy and the balloon just nod your head.

Alright fine. Off to the left, running out into the street where this path out of the park, now a man, a vendor is coming over the lane and he is pushing one of those old-fashioned popcorn wagons. And actually, he has a popper in there which is running on bottled gas and, as he is coming along, the popcorn is spilling out of the popper and down into the glass portion of the cart.

Suddenly the boy sees the popcorn cart and goes running down toward it. When you become **aware** of the popcorn vender and his cart on the path, just nod your head.

Alright fine. Now the boy is running up to the cart, the vendor has stopped and there is the boy looking eagerly up at the popcorn and now you are getting up and walking up over to the cart. And as you do you can feel your mouth watering as you smell, smells like freshly popped corn as you are **aware** of being up close to the cart and having that experience just nod your head.

Fine. And so, you reach in your pocket and you order two boxes of popcorn. And now as you take that popcorn, and you give one box to the boy and kind of indicate that the two of you will walk over to the bench and sit down again just to eat your popcorn. So now you are walking back to the bench and you are sitting down. When you are **aware** that you are seated on the bench with the boy, just nod your head.

Fine. Now he wants, he motions for you to take his balloon so his hands will be free to eat the popcorn. So you just kind of tie the string and the balloon around the end of the bench. And it is bobbing upward.

And now, as the boy eagerly is scooping his hand into the box of popcorn, some of it is spilling over onto the ground. And as you look down, here is a pigeon flying in to pick up some of that popcorn. As you become **aware** of that big pigeon strutting around just nod your head.

And as the boy sees the pigeon he is laughing with delight. Now he takes a hand full of popcorn and throws it out in front of him. And from high up in the tree tops you hear the faint rustling of the leaves. Other birds are coming down. Pigeons and other birds. They are pecking, strutting. The pigeons seem to be strutting as they pick up the popcorn. And now the boy throws out another handful and there is a sudden flurry of wings. And you hear that flurry, as the pigeons swoop up and then down again. As you become **aware** of the pigeons and the flurry of their wings just nod your head.

But now suddenly there is a cry of alarm and the boy is pointing, and it is the balloon. The balloon has become loose and it is floating upward. However, it is kind of lodging. It is getting stuck under the lowest branch and you realize that if you climb up on the bench and you reach up you may be able to catch the string. So now you are climbing up on the bench and you are reaching and straining. As you become **aware** of reaching up to capture that string just nod your head.

Now you have caught it. And now as you bring it down again and hand it to the boy and see his smile suddenly appear through the tears on his cheeks, there is a wonderful feeling of joy and pleasure.

And now there is a calling, a sound. And the boy looks and there is his mother off to the left where the path bends around the shrubbery and she is waving to him and signaling to him to come back to her. As you become **aware** of mother off there on the path nod your head.

So, now the boy in a shy manner but friendly says goodbye, waves, and now he is running off towards his mother, balloon in hand bobbing up and down. And as you see him go you feel a wonderful sense of pleasure and satisfaction over these pleasant and even joyful moments that you have spent here in the park.

Now just let your mind grow clear.

You are **aware** now that you are able to experience a very full, very complete kind of imagery. Including sights, sounds, tastes, feelings. Not just the flat appearance of looking at a picture in a magazine. But you as an organism with special sensory perceptions have been able to fully experience that which I descriptively set out on the canvas for you to respond to.

This time when you open your eyes, you are going to have a much fuller **awareness** of your capability to experience. In fact, you will no longer even need to use the word visualize because you will know it is a word that has the wrong connotations for you. You will know that you are capable of experiencing through all of your senses any time you wish to and any time you need to. And even beyond that from this time forward you will know that you are the architect of your life and that you can set your goals and move toward them at the speed that seems most appropriate for you.

But you now begin to realize that you are unique and there are special things for you to do. Things that can and should be done better by you than by any other person. For never before has life been expressed by any other person in exactly the same way it is now being expressed to you. For if it had been, there would be no use no need for you to be here. And never again will life be expressed in exactly the same way for if it were going to be, there would be no need for you to be here.

So, you think of yourself as a creative person and you now use your great creative power to move toward those goals that will help you to realize your highest potential, which you intuitively perceive.

And that means that you are capable, that you have a way of knowing what you are capable of achieving even though you get to do it. And that is the divine faculty in you and most importantly now I am going to leave you with this realization.

The faculty was given to you for the realization of and the movement towards your goals is your imagination. And your imagination is not just your picture taking or imaging department. It is a vital part of you in which you bring all your sensory responses and most importantly your feelings about yourself and the world about you and your relationship to it. Which is the foundation for the feeling about your ability to be all that you are capable to be.

So you are going to a feel a great sense of confidence and a different perception, because that is what we are dealing with here: **perception**, the way we see things is what determines our lives, determines the nature of our reality. You will feel the sense of being free as if a weight has come off your shoulders, a sense of being free to direct your energy on your own behalf in the manner and form that you decide is best for you.

I am going to slowly count from one to five at the count of five, at the count of five please let your eyelids open, you are calm, rested, refreshed, relaxed and you feel good.

One slowly, calmly, easily, and gently returning to your full awareness once again.

Two each muscle and nerve in your body is loose and limp and relaxed and you feel good.

Three from head to toe you are feeling perfect in every way and

Number four your eyes begin to feel sparkling clear just as though they were bathed in cold spring water. On the next number now eyelids open, fully aware, feeling wonderfully good.

Number five eyelids open now, take a deep breath fill up your lungs and stretch.

Alright let us talk about that.

Conrad: That was, that was a good experience. I liked that. I never trusted it because I could not see it. and uh, that was it, that was the thing that flashed in there that I had it, it was going on and I it was that.
I could not call it up when I needed it. Or maybe I needed it and did not get it or something at times........

Gil: Maybe you were just looking at it the wrong way.

Conrad: Yeah, and there was always something behind. I found out the positive things about not doing it because talking to people that visualize and having that I saw that as being restrictive because it is nice, having a nice clear mind inside, or whatever it is. But I felt as though I was being cheated because I would have the picture.

Gil: And what color was the balloon?

Conrad: Uh, silver.

Gil: (laughter) I never gave it a color

Conrad: Well, I am pretty sure it was.

Gil: Was your popcorn salted?

Conrad: Yeah, laughter. Liked that popcorn.

Observer: Who was the boy with the red hair?

Gil: No, no, that has nothing to do with it. That is, now you get into psychoanalysis, this was not an exercise in psychotherapy evaluation. This was not an experiment in psychoanalytic interpretations.

Conrad: That, that was a good cue, the whole thing was nice, it was okay, it was an it, an enjoyable experience. I liked that. That was better than going to the park and eating popcorn.

Gil: Show your appreciation of this good friend. (applause). You stay for just a moment.
This is a very common mistake and I think it is a mistake for hypnotists to say to people, now I want you to see in your imagination, because many people will have the same feeling. And when you say I want you to visualize, this, the word visualize, for them produces, "but I cannot see anything". Some of them may get up from the session and say to you, well, I could not see anything, some will not bring up that energy to say it to you. Because they feel guilty, they feel disappointed. They say well he expected me to see something and I did not see it. And I do not want to feel guilty so I will just pretend that I saw it.

Instead, do as I did and say, now you are in the park. Put a tree - you notice the difference between put a tree in the park or put a bench, rather than saying I want you to see a bench.

I did not say I want you to see yourself seated on the bench, I said put a person, preferably yourself, on the bench.

Can you see how the avoidance of certain loaded words eliminated the inhibition that had been created by those words, so I hope that that lesson will be meaningful to you and you will avoid telling clients, now I want you to imagine, now I want you to see yourself, now I want you to visualize. And instead, find more creative ways of
doing that, ways that will produce a response instead of a failure.

Until the next time, this is Gil Boyne.

Your Notes

A Variation On Dave Elman's "100, Deeper Asleep" Induction

This is a rather fun way to lead a client into a trance. And yes, it also works like a charm with analytical or untrusting clients.

The induction:

To client:

Please listen carefully:

I will be counting from one hundred down, and after each number, I will say deeper asleep, ninety-nine, deeper asleep, ninety-eight, deeper asleep, and so on.

First, let me lift your right hand like this.
(I am seated at the right side the client, taking and holding their hand by the thumb).
That is right. Just let your arm hang loose and heavy…

Each time I say a number, you will open your eyes, and close them when I say, "deeper asleep". At one point, most likely at 95, maybe 94 you will find your eyelids wanting to stay closed.

Alright, ready?

I then start the countdown slowly, looking at my client, smiling at them as they open and close their eyes, encouraging them at relaxing deeper and deeper each time they close their eyes, *"that is right".*

Your Notes

When it is obvious opening their eyes is getting difficult, I let the client's hand fall on their lap as I say firmly<
"SLEEP"
I then proceed with the work, as usual.

I have also found sometimes holding the client's hand by the thumb is not required.

Using this induction at the second visit of a very stubborn senior client made him go straight into a past life prevalent to the reason he was coming for sessions.

This induction is as easy as it is effective.

Enjoy!

Anny Slegten

Suggestion To Keep A Focus

1-   There is something that you want the pleasure to have.

2-   And from the depth of your being, you are having it right now.

3-   And you may or may not be aware of the fact that what you want to have is inside and outside of your present awareness right now

4-   And what a nice thing to know that you can use both your subconscious mind and conscious mind the pleasure to experience what you want to have, and you are experiencing it right now.

To keep the focus, maintain the feeling in the conversation and keep repeating #1.

Transcript – The Reason Anny Says What She Says.

A Talk During HYP 202 December 6, 2017

As we are going to review it together, I want you to pay attention to the details of it.

I am going to explain to you something extremely important.

Everything you say there has a purpose.
When you look at this you are going to understand something.

That everything I say there is quite a suggestion. Every word of it. For example, when I say,

"…sleep now, this is not the sleep you experience when you fall asleep: I am talking about hypnotic sleep, this means you relax completely your mind and your body so your subconscious mind, free of all restrain is open and receptive to the suggestions you are receiving now."

When you really read that do you realize the suggestion that I had there?

Now, how come I say,

"And during this session the sound of my voice will make you go deeper and deeper into relaxation…".

"During this session every noise that you will hear, during this session...," whatever it is, "

During this session each time I am clearing my throat, you are going twice as deep into relaxation...".

How come I say, "...*during this session...*"?

Each time you are giving a suggestion that is only pertaining to the deepening of the trance you have to put a limit on it. Otherwise, if you do not do that, for example if I had not said, "During this session the sound of my voice will make you go deeper and deeper into relaxation" and then all of a sudden, for example, I am on the radio and they are hearing my voice, what do you think is going to happen?

You must put a limit of any suggestion pertaining at deepening the trance when it is safe for your client to close their eyes.

Therefore, it is *"during this session"* Or, *"As you are listening to this recording, during this recording, the sound of my voice..."* you have to put a time limit on it.

Now, there is something very important about this.

"...and we ask your subconscious mind, open and receptive to the suggestions you are receiving now, to sort all things out, and reveal to you what it feels you should know and understand about the issue that got you here today, and we ask your subconscious mind to reveal it to you in a gentle and most effective manner..."

When you do that, when a client comes in, it does not matter how many times they come in, when the clients come in, they are going to check to make sure you are going to address what they want you to address and not something else. And as long as you do not mention it, they are going to stay on guard.

They are going to relax the moment you say for example,

"…will reveal to you what you should know and understand about you wanting to completely let go of the cigarette", for example.

Or,

"you wanting to slim down",

or whatever it is. When they have an issue, you have to mention it, otherwise they are going to stay on guard because they are afraid you are going to do what you think they should have instead of what they came for.

Question: Would you recommend addressing what they have come in for then right away, in the induction part?

Anny: Well, yes, that is why you have to ask the reason they came for even when they came before,

They do not have to sign the magic paper anymore, they are in the magic chair, and I am taking notes and I say, *"Ok, what do you want today?"*

When they do not know, I put it like that,

"about the issue that got you *here today*.

That is when I do it like that, when they do not know exactly.   *"I know I had to come but I do not know the reason.*

And then, with a smile, I tell them,

"That is fine. How about the priority at subconscious level?"

They do not have to know. Because some people do not know, and say, *"I know I have to come Anny! I know I have to come, but I do not know."*

So, I say, *"It is fine. "*

And how do I get them to go there? You saw me already doing that.

What I do is this. As I let them go into quite a very nice state of relaxation, after the prayer and everything, I said,

"...Contemplate your life, contemplate your life", and if it is for the cigarette I say,

"Contemplate your life, and as you are contemplating your life as you have decided to let go of the cigarette, an emotional feeling is coming up. "

So you know what is the problem.

However, when they do not know what is the problem, I then say to them,

"...as you are there, listening to my voice, going deeper and deeper into that special quality of relaxation, contemplate your life, and as you are contemplating your life, an emotional feeling is coming to you, and when you got it, let me know."

Question: Can you say that one more time?

Anny: When they do not know what it is and it is going to be a priority, at subconscious level priority, when they are really nicely relaxed, after the prayer and everything, I say,
"…contemplate your life, and as you are contemplating your life, an emotional feeling is coming to you and when you got it let me know"

And usually it is something that is pretty sad, and tears are coming up, and I am anchoring I am telling you, and then I say,

"I know you do not like it. I understand you do not like it, the thing is there is a message there, so, just for now, just for now, allow that feeling to come to you, stronger and stronger, just for now, just for now.

And with each exhale, allow that feeling to go back, back, back to whatever it is that started that feeling. Way back. As you get younger and younger."

Now, look at me here. As I say that, I do that to my clients (gestures with hand sliding from head all the way down the client's body).

It is a martial art thing, when they fight, it is a martial art thing, it is a weakening thing (gestures the hand sweeping from the head, down the body) so that they are – weakening their guards.

But the thing is that is my intent!

I want them also to be weaker and as I make this gesture, so that there is a shade there, in front of them (hand would be over the face and moving down over the body).

And I keep saying:

"So, allow. With each inhale allow that feeling to get stronger and stronger, and with each exhale, allow that feeling to go back in time (gesture from face down body) *back in time* (gesture from face down body) *to whatever it is that started that feeling."*

And they go there, let me tell you.

Some people come to feel better and will resist to go to a bad thing.

I catch them anyway.

I say, *"It feels so good* (alright because that is the reason they are there) *that good feeling, let it come to you stronger and stronger,"*

I do the same thing since the good feeling is the bad feeling. *"Let it come stronger and stronger…"* and then I deepen the trance and then I say

"and now…"

I am sneaky, I am not nice and that is ok, it is effective, and so then I say to them, *"Alright, deeper and deeper, it feels so good,"* and I am deepening the trance too at that time, and then, I say,

"Oh, oh, something changed, something changed, it does not feel so good anymore,…" and they go...

Alright?
So, the thing is that some people come to feel better, so they are not going to go back. Well, sorry, you are going to go there.

Now, and when I say, *"Where do you feel it, because an emotional feeling is coming to you, where does it sit in your body?"*

Your Notes

Anny's Teaching

And when they say for example it is here (indicating the chest/heart area) I say, *"Put both hands there, and hold it in a comfortable way to you, there is an emotion there, there is a message there, and it is important for the feeling to know **you know** it is there."*

When they say it is in my head, that is it! You got an analyzer in your chair. And it is no fun. That is ok, you get them anyway.

Question:: Do you deepen the trance then?

Anny: No, I go through the back door.

You know, you have a toolbox, and you can do a whole bunch of things.

Now, also, there is something there that I did not write.

Ok, and I have to get myself in a trance to remember the whole thing…

(three second pause)

there is a time when I go into a trance, that I said,

"As your subconscious mind, open and very receptive to the suggestions you are receiving now, is shifting whatever has to be shifted, improving whatever has to be improved, heal whatever has to be to healed, so that all this, or something even better, now manifests in your attitude, your behaviour, your life in a most pleasant way, and the benefit of this session and the benefit of all the counselling you had prior to this session, will stay with you for hours, days, weeks, months and years to come, much to your surprise and delight."

Now the reason I say, *"… and all the counselling you had prior to this session..."* it is because you know what, I want them to know, that it is ok, to have gone somewhere else before. It really does not matter to me.

That is how come I put that in there. *"…the benefit of this session, and the benefit of all the counselling you had prior to this session, will stay with you."*

Because, even if there was no benefit, according to them, there is something about it, whatever it is. They started a process of looking inside of themselves. It I like having removed some cobwebs and did not get the spider yet. They started their inner work.

Now, sometimes it is not appropriate to say ----, because usually the younger self came up, and they have to make peace with that younger self, let me tell you!

I say to them, *"… and bless each member of your household, bless your family, bless your friends, bless your pets, if you have any, and that includes your house plants, bless your possessions, bless your wishes,…"* And when I know that they have a plan, I would say for example, *"…bless the new project…"* you know. *"…bless the young one that came to you, and bless that younger one, that came to you and helped you today. Bless them and thank them." "Bless your light, that spark of light, that you have within you and thank God, or whoever you perceive God to be, for the wonders of life. You are more relaxed than you have been for a while, and each time you enter this type of relaxation, you will enjoy a deeper and better quality of relaxation."*

Now if you really pay attention to this, you will note that every word I say about this, is quite a suggestion! Although it does not sound that way, it is. Well, it does not sound that way for the client, that is for sure. You people know what I am up to.

Your Notes

Anny's Teaching

You also have to pay attention as how a client feels, not sure of it all,

As I am establishing rapport with a client, smiling, I explain how they are following me in a trance. And they gently follow me in that special quality of relaxation.

Sometimes, I know my client is reluctant to go in a trance, for fear of to go back (regress)in a problem they have caused, feeling a guilty.

I then ask permission to do my work to their benefit.

I explain:

I can do this work very gently, and come for a session once a week for sometimes up to 10 years to resolve what you came here for, or I am going to ask you to help me help you so I can do my work in a more effective way. Your choice.

Your Notes

Canadian Law

(¶ 18-433, A.) **Criminal procedure – Evidence – Refreshing evidence through hypnosis – Accused allowed to testify after memory regained through hypnosis – Evidence admissible as relevant – Hypnosis important factor in determining weight to be given such evidence – Guidelines for use of such evidence.**

The accused was tried for murder and was unable to recall events surrounding the commission of the crime. He regained some memory of those events following hypnosis and the judge allowed him to testify as to those events.

The judge held that the evidence was admissible because it was relevant and that he would provide written reasons for that ruling.

Held: Testimony from a witness whose memory was refreshed through hypnosis was admissible if the evidence was relevant. However, that evidence had to be considered with great caution in order to determine the proper weight to be given to it. The conduct of the hypnotic session had to be carefully examined. Guidelines to minimize the chance that such evidence would be unreliable included, *inter alia*, that the session be conducted by a professional, with only that person and the subject being present, a recording of the session, and a prohibition against suggestive or leading questions. The Court ultimately had to consider all factors in assessing the credibility of the hypnotically induced witness.

R. v. CLARK, May 29, 1984, 32 Alta. L.R. (2d) 353 (Q.B.)

©1984, CCH Canadian Limited

Top Court Bars Use Of Post-Hypnotic Evidence

Updated Thu. Feb. 1 2007 11:01 AM ET

Canadian Press

OTTAWA -- The Supreme Court of Canada has thrown out the use of post-hypnotic evidence in criminal cases, saying the practice is scientifically and legally unreliable.

In a 6-3 decision, the court overturned the second-degree murder conviction of Stephen Trochym, a former Canada Post supervisor from Toronto who was found guilty of killing his former girlfriend.

The ruling means Trochym will get a new trial.

Key evidence in the case came from a woman who testified that she belatedly remembered, after being hypnotized, that she had seen Trochym emerging from the apartment of the victim.

Evidence obtained through hypnosis has been admitted in Canadian courts, under certain circumstances, for some 30 years.

But the Supreme Court majority said the science surrounding the practice is too uncertain, and the dangers of false evidence too great, to continue down that road.

Police can still use hypnosis as an investigative tool, but they will have to obtain other evidence to corroborate any leads they obtain, and can no use the post-hypnotic testimony in court.

Watch the film and listen to Anny's response, when interviewed on CTV regarding

"The Little Warriors"

Ramtha: The Magical Brain – Doorway To A Master's Reality

A transcript of this presentation as well as of two other presentations can be read in:

THE BRAIN – THE CREATOR OF REALITY AND A LOFTY LIFE,

a book published by "North Star Ram".

To purchase the book, visit www.Hun-Nal-Ye.com

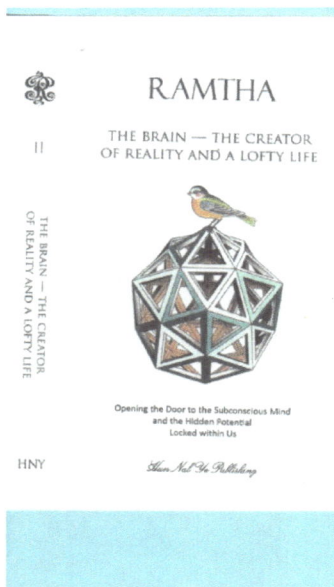

Your Notes

Anny's Teaching

Presenting An Image To The Mid-Brain

First, know what you want the pleasure to have, and/or the result of what you want the pleasure to experience, and see the **result** of what you want to have and/or what you want to experience in your mind.

See it clearly in your mind's eye. Have a clear idea in your mind, something you can **describe**. Make sure it is the **result**. Remember the exercise in HYP 101: What would be different in your life? What would you have that you do not have now? What would you do that you do not do now?

Make sure you are alone in the picture.

Then, close your eyes and **slowly inhale** as you "see" the vision coming to you. Literally see that vision, feel what you want the pleasure to have coming **to you.** Inhale it as if you wanted to swallow it.

Then, as you **slowly exhale**, smile at that vision.

Watch how fast the vision manifests!

Note:

Create only what is in the realm of acceptance.
Remember in HYP 101 what happened with me in North Bay, Ontario?

The Vertigo Induction

This induction was developed by Robert F. Otto, C.HT,
http://robertottohypnosis.com

The International Medical and Dental Hypnotherapist Association

Headquarters:

8852 Sr 3001, Laceyville, Pennsylvania, 18623, U.S.A.
Telephone 570-869-1021   Facsimile 570-869-1249

The Set Up

Okay _____ *(Client's name)*, what I am going to do now is to simply ask you to seat yourself *(suggestion of compliance)* comfortably in the chair. Place your feet so that they do not interfere with any obstructions or touch the floor and place your hands in your lap. *(Make the gesture, unconscious command, of handing them a pen/pencil, or any other appropriate modality)*

After you are comfortably seated, I am going to rotate the chair in a clockwise direction a few times. You will feel a few intermittent interruptions in the rotation as I do this.

However, at some point, you will feel yourself moving in the opposite direction. When this occurs, you will also begin to feel a total and complete sense of total physical relaxation. When you feel yourself moving in that direction, along with physical relaxation, I would like you to simply drop the pen/pencil. The rotation in the opposite direction will become as smooth as silk. A smooth transition.

What I would like you to do with the pen/pencil now is to ask that you direct the pen/pencil to the way you are rotating. When you feel yourself moving to the left, point the pen/pencil to the left. And likewise, when you feel yourself moving to the right, point the pencil to the right. When the rotation becomes as smooth as silk in the opposite direction, drop the pen.

Are you certain that you understand my instructions? Good!

The Induction

Stand behind the client that is safely seated in the chair and place your hands upon their shoulders with slight down pressure. As you do this, speak softly and begin the induction. ***"Just close your eyes now and listen to the sound of my voice. At this time, just relax and ignore any and all outside interference. You are enjoying the feeling of relaxation sweeping over your entire body, from the tips of your toes to the top of your head. Feeling very relaxed and comfortable.***

Take a deep breath in and now out…. Feeling very loose, limp and relaxed in every way".

Begin the rotation….

<u>Additional Instruction for the Therapist.</u>

Rotate the client 8 – 10 times. No more that 13.

After the rotation, allow them to come to a slow and complete stop. Help the stop along if necessary.

As the client comes to a complete stop and the pencil is dropped, begin your favorite deepening technique. Do an arm drop test and begin the session.

From the beginning of the session as the client is seated in the chair to a workable state of hypnosis should range from no more than 25 – 30 seconds before you begin therapy.

Re-affirm the induction immediately after your up count, simply by asking your client how much he enjoyed the "smooth as silk" opposite rotation. *"Smooth as silk, was it?"*

Using a post hypnotic suggestion is beneficial when using the vertigo Induction for demonstration purpose. It gives a clear and concise demonstration that the client was indeed hypnotized!

Unhooking Emotional Hooks

Feeling stuck and unable to move forward?

Here is an exercise I learned from a healer and friend several decades ago. You may record it to monitor yourself through it and remember my choice of words is directly related to the ease of pronunciation....

First, sit in a chair with a straight back.

Now, as you take a slow deep breath, and exhale, put yourself in a hypnotic trance to heighten your state of awareness, same as when we do surrogate sessions.

You know how to do that!

And now, as you take a slow deep breath, and exhale, become aware of your Light, your spark of Life. It is like a mini sun in your chest. Some people can see it, some people can feel it, some people simply know it is there. That Light of yours, that mini sun in your chest, let it shine, let it shine, let it shine in all its might and extend itself at one arm's length above you, beneath you, at each side of you, in front of you and behind you and claim dominion over your space by mentally stating "This my body, this is my space, only Light can come to me, only Light can come from me, only my Light can be here".

And then, as you take another slow deep breath, and exhale, check your aura, the energy field around you and become aware of emotional hooks stuck in your aura, your energy field.

Pause

Unhook every emotional hook stuck in your energy field, keeping you stuck in the situation you are in now, and set yourself free of it all. In your mind perceive them as bungee straps with a hook on each side. As you unhook them, in your mind, perceive them returning to their rightful owners. You will instinctively know who put their emotional hooks on you, and some others you will not.

Pause.

Then check for emotional hooks you put in others' energy field, and retrieve your hooks, setting others free the way you freed yourself.... That is right!

Um, Hum ....

Once done, in your mind, gather your hooks, put them in a box and seal the box.

As you know, there is a lot of energy invested in these emotional hooks. In your mind, write on the side of the box:

To be transformed into self trust, self esteem, awareness of my abilities and strength, enjoying peace of mind (or whatever you want the pleasure to have that energy transformed into**).**

Pause

Once having given precise directions to the energy, in your mind, send the sealed box to the sun to be burned up, consumed, and transformed into what you want. Pay attention to a very powerful feeling in your chest as the energy has been shifted, and breath it in, breath it in, impregnating every cell in your body.

Pause

Your Notes

Anny's Teaching

Now, as you relax more and more, become aware of your aura again, the energy field around you and repair your aura, rearrange it so it is smooth, even, and nice. If some places are torn, in your mind, sew them back with gold thread.

And now, as you are feeling free to move forward, contemplate what you want the pleasure to experience and achieve, and with every breath that you take, going deeper and deeper into a very special quality of relaxation…

Transcript – Guided Self Hypnosis

This was done with a client who explained he used to do self hypnosis years ago to clearly have answers to questions he had in mind, and wanted to experience it again so he could easily practice self hypnosis all by himself.

Anny: All right, first I would like you to think about what do you want to resolve?
Any question in your mind ?
Formulate a question very, very clearly.

What do you want to know? What do you want to resolve? What do you want to accomplish? Just think about it for a moment. Just think about it for a moment. What do you want to know? What do you want to accomplish? What is it?

And as you are contemplating what you want, you are becoming more and more relaxed. More and more at peace.
That is right.

And your breathing becomes more and more relaxed.
That is right.

And as you become more and more relaxed, it is as though everything is slowing down. Slowing down. Slowing down.

And during this experience, the sound of my voice makes you so relaxed, so comfortable and the familiar sounds of the room make you more and more relaxed. More and more at peace and let all your cares fade away. Fade away. Fade away. Fade away.

As I am asking for your protection and your well being and I say:
God, please allow only good thigs to come the person who listens to this recording.

And for this blessing, we give thanks.

And now, become aware of your Light. That Light of yours. That very beautiful light of yours. Let it shine, let it shine. Let it shine throughout every cell of your body, throughout your aura, cleansing your body, cleansing your aura, strengthening your body, and strengthening your aura. Expanding itself at one arm's length above you, beneath you, at each side of you, in front of you and behind you and mentally repeat with me: "This is my body. This is my space. Only light can come to me. Only light can come from me. Only my light can be here.

Slowly inhale and as you slowly exhale, sleep now. Inhale. Slowly exhale. Sleep now. When I say sleep now, this is not the sleep you experience when you fall asleep at night. I am talking about what is called the hypnotic sleep. This means that you relax completely your mind and your body. So your subconscious mind, freed of all restraint, is open and receptive to the suggestions you are receiving during this session.

And during this session, the sound of my voice will make you go deeper and deeper into relaxation,

and also during this session, the familiar sounds of the room make you so relaxed and so comfortable. So relaxed and so comfortable.

And now, as you take a slow deep breath and exhale, I am asking your subconscious mind open and very receptive to the suggestions you are receiving now, to sort all things out and reveal to you whatever it feels you should know and understand about the question, your reason to go into a trance right now.

And I am asking your subconscious mind to reveal it to you at most unexpected time.

It will always be very comforting.
The information will be quite delightful.
And for this blessing, we give thanks.

And now, as you are listening to my voice, going deeper and deeper into that very special quality of relaxation, find yourself at the top of a very beautiful staircase. Absolutely beautiful. It could be indoors; it could be outdoors. A beautiful staircase.

And as you are there, at the top of the staircase, notice how everything looks as you are at the top of it.

And you have one hand on the railing.
That is right.

Notice the feel of the railing under your hand.
That is right.

And notice how you feel deep inside, as you are there standing at the top of the most beautiful staircase.

And as you are standing there, let your quest come to your awareness. Whatever you wanted to accomplish as you are entering this exercise is coming back to mind.

There is something that you want to know. Something that you want to experience. Something you want to resolve. Whatever it is.

And as you are contemplating your quest, you are going down the stairs one step at a time, telling yourself that with each step down, you are going deeper and deeper into relaxation.

And during this session, each time I am clearing my throat you go twice as deep into that very beautiful, very unique quality of relaxation.

And now, as you start to go down the stairs one step at a time, you feel yourself going deeper and deeper in a very beautiful experience of relaxation. Very pleasant, very beautiful experience of relaxation. Going down the steps one step at a time.
That is right.

Feel the steps under your feet. Feel the steps as you are going down the stairs one step at a time.
That is right.
One step at a time. That is right. One step at a time. One step at a time. One step at a time.

And when you are at the bottom of the stairs, sit on the last step.

And become aware of your lungs. Your lungs, they are expanding and contracting, expanding and contracting in a beautiful rhythmic manner and every breath that you take makes you go deeper and deeper and deeper into relaxation. Deeper and deeper. Deeper and deeper into relaxation and as your breath flows, as it comes, as it goes, notice that the sensation is a little cooler when you breath in than when you breath out. Just a little cooler. Just a little cooler.

And as you are sitting there on the last step, in your mind turn around and look at the stairs from the bottom up and notice how the same staircase looks different. And understand that is what life is all about. It is the way we look at it that makes our perception, our reality.

And now in your mind, as you are getting up, you look around and you see a door to a building. In your mind, walk towards it. And when you are there, touch the door. Feel the door. Notice the details of the door and you know that the place it is going to open into is a very special

place. A very special place, totally safe and very beautiful. Safe and beautiful.

So now as you are taking a slow deep breath and as you exhale, open the door. Does it make a sound? Pass through the door. Close the door behind you and turn around.

You will find that there is a mirror there. You could call it a magic mirror.

There was a reason for you to go into this trance. Remember your question. What awareness do you want to have? What do you want to resolve? And now become very much aware of how you feel as you walk towards that very, very special mirror.

And as you are standing now in front of what one could call the magic mirror, look into it and you realize that the mirror is, in fact, a door to another world where everything you want to know is answered.

Enjoy it and most of all; trust the awareness that is coming to you.
And become very much aware of how you feel as that awareness is coming to you.
And know that you are safe. Trust the information. Trust the awareness. Welcome the events.

As you are experiencing the awareness, you realize that you can come back to this very special place any time you want to.

And when you are satisfied with the awareness, thank it to have come.

Embrace the awareness and leave the place and come back to what is called full awareness, feeling relaxed, renewed, retaining the information and being totally at peace with yourself and with the world around you.

Having learned something.
Having learned the importance of totally, totally trusting yourself.

Trust yourself. Trust the awareness that came to you.
Trust it. Welcome it. And embrace it, remembering that you can visit this place again anytime you want to.

And now as you have experienced whatever you want to experience from the depth of your being, you can at will leave the room and come back to what is called full awareness, feeling refreshed, relaxed, renewed.
Remembering clearly the experience and feeling at peace with yourself and with the world around you.

And now I am going to count from 1 to 5 and I will say:
Your eyes are open. You are fully aware. Feeling refreshed, relaxed, renewed.
Totally, totally at peace with yourself and with the world around you.

One, slowly, calmly, easy, gently, beginning to return to full awareness once again. Enjoying a sharp mind, a clear head and a tranquil heart.

Two, each muscle and nerve in your body is loose, limp, relaxed and you feel wonderfully good.
You feel at peace with yourself and with the world around you.
Enjoying a sharp mind, a clear head and a tranquil heart.

Three, from head to toe you are feeling so much better in every way.
Physically better. Mentally better. Emotionally cool, calm and serene.
Enjoying a sharp mind, a clear head and a tranquil heart.

Four, your eyes begin to feel sparkling clear as bathed in cool spring water.

Five, eyelids open. Open your eyes. You are fully aware. Take a slow deep breath. Open your eyes and give yourself a very good stretch.

Your Notes

Client's feedback:

Anny: What surprised you?

Client: It went to the heart of the matter.

Anny: What?

Client: I say, it went right to the heart of the matter.

Anny: Good.

Client: Yes, it is free, emotionally.

Anny: That is okay. Allow it to happen. Just allow the emotions. Just allow it.

Client: I never relax. My body was like taught the whole time. Except for my lower – my arms.

Anny: Yes, that is because you are not used to relaxing, I suppose.

Client: Probably.

Anny: Also, there is one thing that, with hypnosis, you become very much aware of your body. So, you become aware of something and what is nice is that you are.

You know I stopped your recording here, so it is mine only that is going or is still on. So only that experience will be on your r4ecording. Nothing else. What we say now is not on your recording at all.

It is quite amazing that as you learn to become more and more relaxed, you are going to allow your body to go to that level. It is an allowing.

Client: I am not a visualizer.

Anny: Well, some people do and some people do not. It is a knowing.

Client: I say I am kinaesthetic.

Anny: Yes, so am I.

Client: And that is overwhelming. I did not actually see the mirror, but I knew it was there. And then I knew I was there and I was in the forest. I did not see any trees, but I knew they were there. I went by a porch with a rocking chair. But I could fly in a circle. It was quite peaceful, and it was very loving.

Anny: Did you get what you came here for today?

Client: I was not expecting this.

Anny: You were not expecting this.?

Client: Of course, I am a control person.

Anny: That is okay, that is how come your body is tense like that.

Client: I am amazed that I am aware at all times. It is like watching a movie where you can sense that now. It would be nice to visualize.

Anny: You know what, we all visualize. It is a knowing. It is not like seeing on TV. It is a knowing.

Client: But you know sometimes I dream and I know I am in a different place and the colours are glowing. People are glossing - it is like a glossy people's page, where the people are more beautiful than that. The colours are so outstanding.

Anny: It is although you do not see it, you can describe it.

Client: Yes, I did see colours were really, really vivid, but they never seem to blend into other things. They were very stark.

Anny: We are all different in the way we visualize. It is a knowing.

Client: But I do - I am a negative hallucinator - at least I read that. Where I can say look at that brass - the brass handles and they would disappear, but I would not see the holes where they were. They would disappear and I could just see the wood. I sit in my living room and they all disappear.

Anny: Remember something, you begin to wonder what is reality and what is illusion.

Client: Yes, like when I read _____ Watson. He said he had a little girl there that made everything disappear. The trees and everything. So it is a world of reality. If you believe it, it is there. If you do not – it is not there.

Anny: Exactly, that is why some people do not see anything. They blank it out.

Client: But that was amazing.

Anny: That is it for today.

Client: Thank you

Transcript – Self Confidence

Sitting in the recliner, the client was looking at a year
calendar on the wall. Everything colour coded.

Anny: Okay, thank you. All the thoughts about what I am doing, so I do
not think of it that way.

Okay that is hypnosis (yellow), that is Reiki (blue), that is courses I am
taking (orange).

Gerry: Well, that is good.

Anny: That is time off (green).

Gerry: No that is good. I know people who are organized, but I would
be – you would be very organized.

Anny: Well, thank you!

Gerry, I learned through the years that when I use a technique called
anchoring during hypnotherapy session, the session is faster, smoother,
much more comfortable for my client and we come to a closure so much
faster.

Gerry: Okay.

Anny: Anchoring can be used in many ways and the way I use it, I will
be touching your knees and it will be a firm touch like that.

Gerry: Okay.

Anny: Sometimes I will touch this knee. Sometimes the other.
Sometimes both and I would like to have your permission to do so.

Gerry: Okay.

(Testing client to establish what technique to use)

Anny: Okay. So now, first things first, how do you feel right now?

Gerry: Oh, I feel fine. I feel relaxed and comfortable.

Anny: I notice that you are quite tall. Do you want a cushion behind your neck or is it fine?

Gerry: I think I can kind of settle into this. Yes, I feel pretty comfortable. Yes.

Anny: All right. Okay, now have you been hypnotized before that you are aware of?

Gerry: No.

Anny: Not that you are aware of. All right, well you know, let us say you are reading a book and you are really into the book. You are really enthralled by the story.

You are in the book and you are totally there, although you know which room you are in. You do not pay too much attention about what is going on, but you know who is there, who is talking. You answer, without really knowing what the people ask, you know. It is about the same thing. There is a journal about you inside of you.

Gerry: Okay.

Anny: And, there is something about whatever you have that confidence issue here. You know what, it has reason. There is a reason for you to be that way and deep down you know it.

And I am using hypnosis so you stay conscious as you go to check out the story inside of you. That is what I want, so that you realize what is going on with you there, how come you are like that and then you can change whatever you want to change.

Gerry: Okay.

Anny: You are in full control of that.

Gerry: Okay, good.

Anny: Okay. Yes, you are in full control of that. So, stare at my fingers Gerry. Stare at my fingers and listen to my voice. Keep your gaze on my fingers and listen to my voice. Your eyelids are getting so heavy, so heavy.

Take a slow deep breath Gerry and as you exhale, close your eyes and enjoy that feeling of relaxation that is coming upon you each time you close your eyes.

That is right.

And the familiar sounds of this room make you so relaxed. So comfortable. So relaxed. So comfortable.

And during this experience each time you close your eyes, you will go deeper and deeper in a very pleasant state of re-lax-a-tion.

So, at the count of three, open your eyes.

One, two, three.

Stare at my fingers and listen to my voice.
Keep your gaze on my fingers and listen to my voice.
Your eyelids are getting so heavy, so heavy, so heavy.

Take a slow deep breath and as you exhale, close your eyes and enjoy the experience. Enjoy the re-lax-a-tion.

That is right.

Enjoy the relaxation.
It is if though everything is slowing down, everything is slowing down.

That is right.

(Creating Eye Catalepsy)

So now you will find that your eyelids are getting rather heavy, so heavy, so heavy.

That is right and you will notice how heavy your eyelids are when on the count of three, you will try to open them.

So: one, two, three, try to open your eyes.
That is right. That is right.

So take a slow deep breath and as you exhale, just enjoy the relaxation and let all your cares fade away, fade away, fade away, fade away.

As I am asking for your protection and your well being and I say, dear God, please allow only good things to come to Gerry and Anny, the hypnotherapist, and for this blessing we give thanks.

And now you ask to be placed into the protection of your very own light. Your very own light, your spark of life. It is like a mini sun in your chest.

Some people can see it, some people can feel it, some people simply know it is there.

That light of yours, that very beautiful light of yours, let it shine, let it shine, let it shine throughout every cell of your body, throughout your aura.

Cleansing your body, cleansing your aura. Strengthening your body, strengthening your aura.

Extending itself at one arm's length above you, beneath you, at each side of you, in front of you and behind you and mentally repeat with me:

> This is my body, this is my space.
> Only light can come to me.
> Only light can come from me.
> Only my light can be here.

Slowing inhale and as you slowly exhale, sleep now.
Inhale. Slowly exhale. Sleep now.

When I say, sleep now, this is not the sleep you experience when you fall asleep at night. I am talking about what is called the hypnotic sleep. This means that you relax completely your mind and your body, so your subconscious mind freed of all restrain is open and receptive to the suggestions you are receiving during this session.

(Installing a limit to the suggestion pertaining to the deepening the trance)

And **during this session**, the sound of my voice will make you go deeper and deeper into relaxation.

During this session, each time I am touching one of your knees, you will go twice as deep into relaxation.

And **during this session**, the sound of my voice will make you go deeper and deeper into relaxation.

During this session, each time I am touching one of your knees, you will go twice as deep into relaxation.

And also **during this session**, each time the ventilation system is going on and off, on and off, you will go so much deeper, so much deeper into relaxation. Deeper and deeper, deeper and deeper into relaxation and let all your cares fade away fade away, fade away, fade away.

And as you take a slow deep breath, and exhale, going deeper and deeper in that wonderful state of relaxation, enjoying it more and more, **during this session** the familiar sounds of this room make you go deeper and deeper and deeper into relaxation. Letting all your cares fade, fade away, fade away.

And as you take a slow deep breath, and exhale, contemplate your confidence issue.

And as you are contemplating your confidence issue, there is a feeling about the whole thing that is coming to you. A very uncomfortable feeling as you are contemplating your confidence issue.

Just contemplate it and become very much aware of that very uncomfortable feeling that is coming to you and pay attention to your body as that issue is coming to you.

Feel your body and become very much aware of where there is a feeling sitting in your body. Where is it sitting in your body? Where is it sitting in your body?

Gerry: My stomach.

Anny: Yes. Put your hands on it and make sure you are comfortable. That is right.

That uncomfortable feeling, it is in the stomach. In the stomach. That is right, it is in your stomach.

And as you take a slow deep breath and exhale, with your mind go into that feeling right here.

Go into it and there is something about it. How old are you when you have that feeling deep inside?

How old are you in that feeling?

Gerry: I am not sure.

Anny: If you were sure, what would it be? Trust it. Even if it does not make sense to you, when you feel that way deep inside, how old are you? Trust what comes.

Gerry: Six.

Anny: You are six years old. Now six years old Gerry. Can you see a little Gerry at six. Do you remember a picture of you at six or can you feel yourself, the way you felt at six years old?

Gerry: Um humm. Yes.

Anny: Yes, what? Which one?

Gerry: I can see a picture of myself.

Anny: You see a picture of yourself. With your other hand, in your mind, hold that Picture of you at six years old.

A six year old little boy was feeling that way right there and as you are looking at the picture and feeling the way the little boy, the young boy is feeling, you will become very much aware of what is going on.

That six year old Gerry has such an uncomfortable feeling. Right there in his stomach. What is going on?
Trust what comes.

Gerry: I'm ….

Anny: Trust what comes.

Gerry: I am staying at a friend's house.

(Repeat your client to stay in your client's mode)

Anny: You are staying at a friends house,

and what is happening that six year old Gerry has an uncomfortable feeling.
 He is staying at a friend's house and? And what happened next?

Gerry: Well I do not know what is going on.

Anny: Umm humm. You do not know what is going on, and?

Gerry: And I am lonely because I am away from my family.

Anny: And you are lonely, okay. You do not know what is going on. And you are lonely because you are away from your family.

Very good. You understand that six year old is feel, don't you?

Gerry: Umm humm.

Anny: Umm humm.

Make sure that whatever way you feel is the right way to do it, that six year old knows that you understand.

And what is happening next?
What is happening?
What is next?
What is happening next?

Gerry: Uhummm.

Anny: Or ask six year old Gerry. Here he is, he is feeling uncomfortable. There is an uncomfortable feeling in his stomach.
He is staying at a friend's house.
He does not know what is going on, lonely because he is away from his family, therefore…?

Trust what comes.
There is a six year old there that feels so uncomfortable. He feels so uncomfortable. He is away from his family, therefore….. therefore ….

Gerry: I feel, I feel just lonely and empty.

Anny: Lonely and empty.

Take a slow deep breath Gerry and as you exhale, from the bottom of your heart explain to little Gerry what happened. The first thing you will do though, is asking him to have a look at you.
Does he know that you are 40 now?

Gerry: Ummm humm.

Anny: And explain to him what happened. Six years old. Do you know what happened that he got there at a friend's house?

Gerry: Ummm humm.

Anny: So explain it to him. Explain it to him.

Gerry: Well your Mom and Dad had to leave because your Dad had to go to the hospital and you had to stay behind because you are in school.

Anny: Did he see his Dad again?

Gerry: Ummm humm.

Anny: And how did he feel when he could see his Dad again.

Gerry: Ohhh, happy.

Anny: He was happy. Yes. He was happy.
Breath in that happiness. He could see his Dad again. Just breath in that feeling. Breath in that feeling.

And as you take a slow deep breath and exhale, together with six year old Gerry, you are going to go back and forth in time, back and forth, back and forth to feeling the same way in another situation.

Feeling the same way in another situation and when you got it, let me know. Same feeling. Allow the feeling to go wherever it wants to go.

The same feeling, another situation.

Gerry: Ummm, in school.

Anny: What happened in school? How old is Gerry?

Gerry: Six.

Anny: Six again. Umm, okay. In school, what is happening in school that little Gerry is feeling that way?

Gerry: Umm, I am in class.

Anny: Umm hum And what is happening?

Gerry: I am, I am sitting in class

Anny: And…

Gerry: I am **feeling bad.**

Anny: Feeling bad?

Gerry: Uhhh huh.

Anny: What is happening that six year old Gerry is sitting in class feeling bad?

Gerry: Uhhh, because this kid knows that my Dad died.

Anny: And, kids know and what is happening?

Gerry: Ummm, awww, I feel embarrassed because I am different.

Anny: Feeling embarrassed because you are different.
What is it that you are different?

Gerry: Because I do not have a Father.

Anny: Ummm humm.
And… ?
Feeling different, embarrassed, you do not have a Father.
And…?

Your Notes

Gerry: Also, I miss my Father.

Anny: I did not get that.

Gerry: I miss …

Anny: Of course.
And … ?
Gerry: I am sad because I miss my Dad.

Anny: Ummm humm.

Gerry: So it…

Anny: And what comes next? … What comes next? …
What comes next? …
What comes next? …
You missed your Dad.
And…?
How is six year old feeling about the whole thing?

Gerry: Lonely.

Anny: Lonely.

Gerry: Unsure.

Anny: Unsure.
Now there is something about the whole thing.

So as you take a slow deep breath and exhale, go deeper and deeper into relaxation. Deeper and deeper, deeper and deeper and I would like to compare the feelings little Gerry had at six years old when all that was happening. Compare it to the feelings you have now.

When you want to socialize, meet people, meet outside of work, just socialize,

I would like you to compare the feelings of the six year old to the feelings you have now.

When you are, you want – you do not feel confident at all, socializing, meeting people, meeting women.

There is something about it and I would like you to compare the two feelings.

And then give me the result of that comparison.

Gerry: It feels the same.

Anny: It feels the same.

All right, so take a slow deep breath and exhale.

Go back to the six year old. Go back to him and explain to him that here you are 34 years later, still feeling the same way.

(Deepening the trance)

So, as you take another deep breath and exhale, become aware of your lungs.

Your lungs, they are expanding and contracting, expanding and contracting in a beautiful rhythmic manner and every breath that you take makes you go deeper and deeper and deeper into relaxation.

And as your breath flows, as it comes, as it goes, notice that the sensation is a little cooler when you breath in than when you breath out.

Just a little cooler. Just a little cooler.

So as you take a slow deep breath and exhale, connect with the six year old and as you are explaining to him that here you are 34 years later feeling the same way, ask him to go back and forth in your life with you, back and forth, back and forth.

And what is he trying to convey as he is feeling that way?
What is he using it for? What is he using it for?

Trust what comes.

Gerry: He is trying to protect himself.

Anny: Okay he is using it to protect himself. Protect himself from what?

Gerry: Ummm, from being hurt.

Anny: Okay, from being hurt. Do you understand that?

Gerry: Ummm, yes.

Anny: Okay, you are talking from the six year old point of view. Can you understand that?

Gerry: Ummm, not really, no.

Anny: No, what is it that you are not understanding from the six year old point of view that he would use that to protect him from being hurt?

Gerry: I am not sure.

Anny: Okay.

So now as you take a slow deep breath and exhale, I would like you to go back and forth in your life with six year old.

Take him by the hand and go back and forth in your life and notice how wanting to protect yourself created – what it created, by doing that to protect yourself – the other side of the coin.

And when you are finished let me know.
Just make him aware of that.

Become very much aware of the other side of the coin.
By using that to protect yourself, what did you create? (music)
What did you create?

Gerry: I don't know.

Anny: Well, what is your reason to be here today?
What is the other side of the coin?
Are you understanding something there?

Gerry: No.

Anny: Compare the feelings you have. That became a confidence issue when you want to socialize and everything, Compare it to the feelings of the six-year-old. He explained to you that he developed it to protect himself from being hurt.

But then, by doing that, what did he create?

How do you feel?
You want to meet people and there is that feeling that comes up…

Gerry: Ummmm hummm.

Anny: So what is the other side of the coin?

I am going to give you an analogy that is particular – that way you use that feeling, that attitude or behavior, you use it to protect yourself from being hurt. It is like putting a fence around you. If you put a fence around you, you protect yourself from the exterior. And on the other hand, you cut yourself off too, don't you?

Gerry: Ummm humm.

Anny: So have a look at the two sides of the coin.

With that attitude that you started to protect yourself as a little boy because you felt lonely, embarrassed, missing your Dad.

Gerry: Ummm humm.

Anny: So you put a fence around you with that, don't you?

Gerry: Ummm humm.

Anny: But then, what is the other side of it?

Gerry: There is no happiness.

Anny: No happiness.

Gerry: No joy.

Anny: No joy.

Gerry: No love.

Your Notes

Anny: No love, Yes. So what would you like to have now in your life, now that you are 40?

Gerry: Love and happiness.

Anny: Feeling safe at meeting people.

Gerry: Yes.

Anny: Totally trusting your intuition too and knowing when it is very, very safe to do it and also when it is safer to abstain from that relationship.

 Do you understand what I am saying there?

Gerry: No.

Anny: That you have to use your own judgement there.

 At the moment you are on full automatic, responding from a six year old point of view. Automatically you put a fence around you.

Gerry: Ummm hummm.

Anny: Now, you are about to make an opening in the fence now, are you not?

Gerry: Ummm humm.

Anny: Yes, so allow life to come to your life really. Allow love to come into your life too. Since you are very good at designing, playfully with little Gerry, find a way to explain how with graphics or putting plastics around you, whatever. Find a way to explain how having done that because he felt so lonely. He missed his Dad, felt different. How he built a fence around himself.

By the way, because at six years old, you were quite small, find yourself on the ground. Show him that because for him the fence was higher, right?

So you sit down on the ground as he is standing next to you and show him the fence he built around himself.

And when you are finished, let me know.

Gerry: Okay.

Anny: So now, stand up and pick the little boy in your arms so that his eyes are at your eyes level, as you are standing now at 40 years old.

And look where the fence is – how high is the fence now?
And as you are holding the little boy in your arms, let him look over the fence.

Gerry: Ummm humm.

Anny: How does it feel Gerry?

Gerry: Good.

Anny: It feels good. So now, what do you want to do, so that you can allow love to come into your life, happiness and joy?

What are you going to do with that fence?

Ask the little boy to grow up, or what? Or put a gate in the fence?

Gerry: Knock it down.

Anny: All right. How do you feel about doing that?

Gerry: I would like to.

Anny: Well, how is the six year old feeling about that?

Gerry: He would like to.

Anny: He would like to.

All right take a breath Gerry and as you exhale, together with six year old, knock down the fence. And when you are finished let me know.

Gerry: Okay.

Anny: So now, take a deep breath and as you exhale, together with six year old Gerry, advance into the future.

See yourself first at work, feeling so much more comfortable.

And as you take a slow deep breath and exhale, together with six year old Gerry, enjoy the new freedom at being able to socialize. Enjoy the new freedom. Enjoy it.

(Collapsing the anchors)

And breath in that new freedom.
Just breath it in.
Just breath it in.

As something inside of you is shifting.
And the shift is steady and progressive.
So smooth, so progressive that it will feel totally, totally comfortable to you.

So now, in your mind, go to the beginning of all this and when you are there, simply nod.

Do you remember how that attitude started about socializing and being with others ?

Go back there, together with six year old Gerry and when you are there, simply nod.

Thank you.

(Time line.)

Now, together with six year old Gerry, advance to what was the middle of the whole thing. It could be what became the most painful situation because of it and when you are there, simply nod.

Thank you.

And now as you take a slow deep breath and exhale, you are going to advance to the end of it. When the shift inside of you has happened…

It could be today, tomorrow, the 15th of February … I have no idea. Advance to when the whole thing has settled down within you.

As your subconscious mind open and very receptive to the suggestions you are receiving now is sorting all things out will reveal to you whatever else it feels you should know and understand.

As your subconscious mind is making all the necessary improvements right now so that all this or something even better now manifests itself in your attitude, your behavior, your life. The joy of it. In a most delightful way.

And the benefits of this session and the benefits of all the counselling that you had prior to this session will stay with you for hours, days, weeks, months and years to come.
And so it is. And so it is. And so it is. And so it is.

<u>Suggestion For A Good Night Sleep</u>

And tonight, and every night when you are ready to fall asleep with your head on your pillow, remember how you feel right now. Remember being in this office, in this chair.

Remember the sound of my voice and then you will take a slow deep breath and as you exhale, you will close your eyes and go into a wonderful slumber.

As your subconscious mind is sorting all things and will improve whatever it feels can be improved. So that you can live fully, physically, emotionally, mentally and spiritually.

To wake up a minute or two before waking up time, feeling refreshed, relaxed, renewed, totally, totally at peace with yourself and with the world around you.

That is right and so it is.

And now, I am going to count from one to five and then I will say, your eyes are open. You are fully aware. Very refreshed, relaxed, renewed, totally, totally at peace with yourself and with the world around you. Enjoying a sharp mind, a clear head and a tranquil heart.

One, slowly, calmly, easy, gently, beginning to return to full awareness once again. Enjoying a sharp mind, clear head and a tranquil heart.

Two, each muscle and nerve in your body is loose, limp, relaxed and you feel wonderfully good. You feel at peace with yourself and with the world around you, enjoying a sharp mind, a clear head and a tranquil heart.

Three, from head to toe, you are feeling so much better in every way. Physically better, mentally better, emotionally cool, calm and serene. Enjoying a sharp mind, a clear head and a tranquil heart.

Four, your eyes begin to feel sparkling clear as you bath it in cool spring water.

And now five, eyelids open, open your eyes. You are fully aware Gerry. Take a slow deep breath. Fill up your lungs and give yourself a pretty good stretch.

Come on!

Gerry: Okay.

Anny: What surprised you the most?

Gerry: Surprised me the most? Well, I am not sure.

Anny: Okay, that is fair enough. If you were sure, what would it be?

Gerry: Well, I am not, I am not… I do not think I was really surprised.

Anny: Okay, fair enough. What came to your awareness that you could join together this time around?

Gerry: What am I more aware of right now?

Anny: When you review the whole thing?

Gerry: That at such a young age, that kind of feeling and attitude started at such an age.

Anny: It always starts, usually, not always then, and usually it is very young. Um hum.

Understand that at that age it was the only coping mechanism. You must understand that. From six year old, there is all that stuff going on. That was the only way he could cope.

Gerry: Uhh huh. I don't – one thing I really wonder about right now is if I really found the right or if that was really the right.

Anny: Okay, then the only way to find that out is to live. You will know. Some people the shift is like that. Sometimes the shift takes about two weeks. Because then it is smoother and looks more normal, so to speak, than it is overnight.

Gerry: Oh yes.

Anny: Okay, overnight, everybody is going to say, ohhh. But if it is over a period of a week or two, then the transition is so smooth that even you will no really realize what is going on. And so, I know that from what happened here. So, give yourself a week or two to know and you will know.

Yes, you will know. Ummhumm.

Transcript – Recording For Surgery Pauline

Alright, please make yourself as comfortable as possible. And make sure you are in a place where it is safe for you to close your eyes, and as you take a slow, deep breath, and exhale, close your eyes.

And become aware of your lungs. Your lungs: they are expanding and contracting, expanding and contracting, in a beautiful, rhythmic manner, and every breath that you take, makes you go deeper and deeper and deeper into relaxation. And as your breath flows, as it comes, as it goes, notice that the sensation is a little cooler when you breathe in than when you breathe out. Just a little cooler. Just a little cooler. And let all your cares fade away, fade away, fade away.

As I am asking for our protection and our wellbeing, and I say, "God, please allow only good things to come to Pauline and me Anny, the hypnotherapist.

And for this blessing, we give thanks.

And now, you ask to be placed into the protection of your very own light, your very own light, your spark of life, it is like a mini sun in your chest. Some people can see it, some people can feel it. Some people simply know it is there.

That light of yours, that very beautiful light of yours, let it shine, let it shine. Let it shine throughout every cell of your body, throughout your aura, cleansing your body, cleansing your aura, strengthening your body, strengthening your aura, extending itself at one arm's length above you, beneath you, at each side of you, and behind you, and mentally repeat with me.

This is my body. This is my space. Only light can come to me, only light can come from me, only my light can be here.

And as you take a slow, deep breath and exhale, listen to my voice, only to my voice. You know that this is a guided hypnosis recording. You know how effective and powerful hypnosis is. So enjoy listening to it, as your subconscious mind is getting the message, loud and clear.

Trust the people, trust the surgeon, and trust also your decision to have that surgery. You know it is for you to be very much more comfortable in your body, from the top of your head, to the tip of your toes. And you know also, how good it is to be able to just relax, breathe easily, knowing that with each exhale, your body, your lungs are flushing out whatever has to be flushed out of your body. That is right, you know that. As you go deeper and deeper into relaxation, you trust the surgeon at doing the surgery correctly and efficiently.

So just take a slow, deep breath, and as you exhale, relax, trusting the surgeon, and trusting also your subconscious mind. Your subconscious mind knows very well that during surgery whatever is said, during surgery by the surgery personnel pertains to themselves and to them alone. As you are going deeper and deeper into a wonderful state of relaxation.

Your body knows what to do to heal. And it is starting to heal, the moment the surgery has started. Your body knows exactly what to do. So relax, relax your subconscious mind is doing its job. As you are relaxed like that, allow yourself to become comfortable from the top of your head, to the tip of your toes. And having great pleasure in functioning normally, physically, mentally, and emotionally, spiritually and financially.
That is right.

And your body knows what to do. It knows that with each exhale, your body is releasing whatever is to be released. Breathing easily, breathing very easily, that is right. And as you are there, listening to my voice, going deeper and deeper into relaxation, you know how hypnosis is powerful,

and you also know that your subconscious mind is open and very receptive to the suggestions you are receiving, that is right. So take a slow, deep breath again, and as you gently exhale, your subconscious mind knows exactly what to do so that you will breathe really easily. So easily, it is so easy that the surgery feels very benign. It is just a little thing, it is so easy to breathe. And you feel very comfortable too, very, very comfortable, from the top of your head to the tip of your toes. Very comfortable in your skin, functioning well.

Your subconscious mind also knows what to do for you to heal quickly and perfectly.

That is right. It is such a calm, fine feeling, going into another state of awareness, becoming very deeply relaxed, allowing your body to regulate itself to very good health.

That is right. Allowing your body to regulate itself to very good health, in a very pleasant, and natural manner. Your body knows what to do, to heal quickly.

That is right. To heal very quickly and well. Your body knows what to do to breathe easily. That is right. And your body knows exactly what to do to move easily.
So relax, relax, and as you take a slow, deep breath, and exhale, see yourself walking, breathing, happy to be alive.

Very, very, very comfortable in your body, from the top of your head to the tip of your toes. Very, very comfortable. So relax, trust your decision to have that surgery. Trust the surgeon, and most of all, trust your subconscious mind. It knows exactly what to do. And trust your body to respond perfectly, heal quickly and comfortably. And you feel so relaxed, so comfortable. Having great, great pleasure at feeling great and looking great too. Feeling great, and looking great too. That is right. Looking really great. Feeling comfortable. Feeling really good in your skin. And for this blessing, we give thanks.

And now that Light of yours, that very beautiful Light of yours, make it shine. Wrap it up, so to speak, allow it to shine in all its might, and direct that Light of yours throughout your body, to flush out whatever has to be flushed out, and send it to the sun, to be burnt up, consumed and transformed, into something very, very beneficial to you. Feeling so great.

So give the Light a job, what do you want the Light to do? You want to be fine, safe, in very good health, from the top of your head to the tip of your toes. And for this blessing, we both give thanks.

So relax, your subconscious mind got the message; it knows what to do. It knows what you want. You want to breathe easily, that is right. And to feel great and be able to move, and function normally. That is right. You want to be able to talk as much as you want. That is right. You want to feel comfortable in your body, from the top of your head, to the tip of your toes.

And your subconscious mind got the message, loud and clear, to put a kind of a shield, during surgery, a kind of a shield, so that whatever is talked about by the surgery personnel is bounced back to them, because it pertains to them. That is right. And a safety zone is being built around you. And for this blessing, we give thanks.

So, allow yourself to take a slow, deep breath, and as you exhale, just slide back, slide back into a wonderful state of relaxation, that is right. Just relax. Relax. Relax. Relax. And for this blessing, we give thanks.

And the benefit of this recording and the benefit of all the counseling you had prior to this recording, will stay with you for hours, days, weeks, months, and years to come. And so it is. And so it is. And so, take a slow, deep breath, and as you exhale, just allow it. Allow yourself to go deeper, and deeper, and deeper into relaxation.

And have wonderful dreams, wonderful dreams. To come back a minute or two before the time established for you to come back to full awareness,

feeling relaxed, refreshed, renewed, at peace with yourself and the world around you, ready for a wonderful experience. It is so great to be alive. Breathing easily. Speaking easily. Moving easily and comfortably. And so it is. And so it is.

So, just sleep now, just sleep now. Sleep now. And as you take a slow, deep breath and exhale, going deeper and deeper into that wonderful state of relaxation, realize that there is a twin like you somewhere in an alternate dimension, who is looking at you now, smiling and doing whatever has to be done, so that this experience is the most gratifying and beneficial experience for you. Feeling totally, totally at peace.

Breathing easily
talking easily, moving easily, even thinking easily. Feeling totally, totally at peace with yourself and with the world around you. So sleep now, sleep now. You are in very, very good hands.

Be at peace with yourself. Be totally, totally, at peace with yourself, and with the world around you. Life is great. Life is totally great. Physically, emotionally, mentally, spiritually and financially.

And so it is. And so it is.

www.success-and-more.com

www.success-and-more.com

www.success-and-more.com

www.success-and-more.com

www.success-and-more.com

www.success-and-more.com

www.success-and-more.com

www.success-and-more.com

www.success-and-more.com

www.success-and-more.com

www.success-and-more.com

www.success-and-more.com

www.success-and-more.com

www.success-and-more.com

www.success-and-more.com

www.success-and-more.com

www.success-and-more.com

www.success-and-more.com

www.success-and-more.com

www.success-and-more.com

www.success-and-more.com

www.success-and-more.com

www.success-and-more.com

www.success-and-more.com

www.success-and-more.com

www.success-and-more.com

www.success-and-more.com

www.success-and-more.com

www.success-and-more.com

www.success-and-more.com

www.success-and-more.com

www.success-and-more.com

www.success-and-more.com

www.success-and-more.com

www.success-and-more.com

www.success-and-more.com

www.success-and-more.com

www.success-and-more.com

www.success-and-more.com

www.success-and-more.com

www.success-and-more.com

Online Store, Contact, And More…

You may contact Anny by visiting any of her websites and scroll down the home page to the contact information.

http://www.annyslegten.com
Anny's private website and online store.

http://www.success-and-more.com
To find the description of the many services offered, and more.

http://www.htialberta.com
The Hypnotism Training Institute of Alberta including descriptions of hypnosis and hypnotherapy courses given.

http://www.reiki-canada.com
About the Reiki Training Centre of Canada.

http://www.slegtenianhypnosis.com
Although open to anyone interested in this fascinating hypnosis modality, this website information is for graduates of the Hypnotism Training Institute of Alberta.

http://www.connectwithanny.com
This is the best place to keep up to date with Anny – including seeing all her latest books and how to order them on Amazon.

Other Books By Anny Slegten…

REIKI PURE AND SIMPLE

Volume I: The Sacred Rites

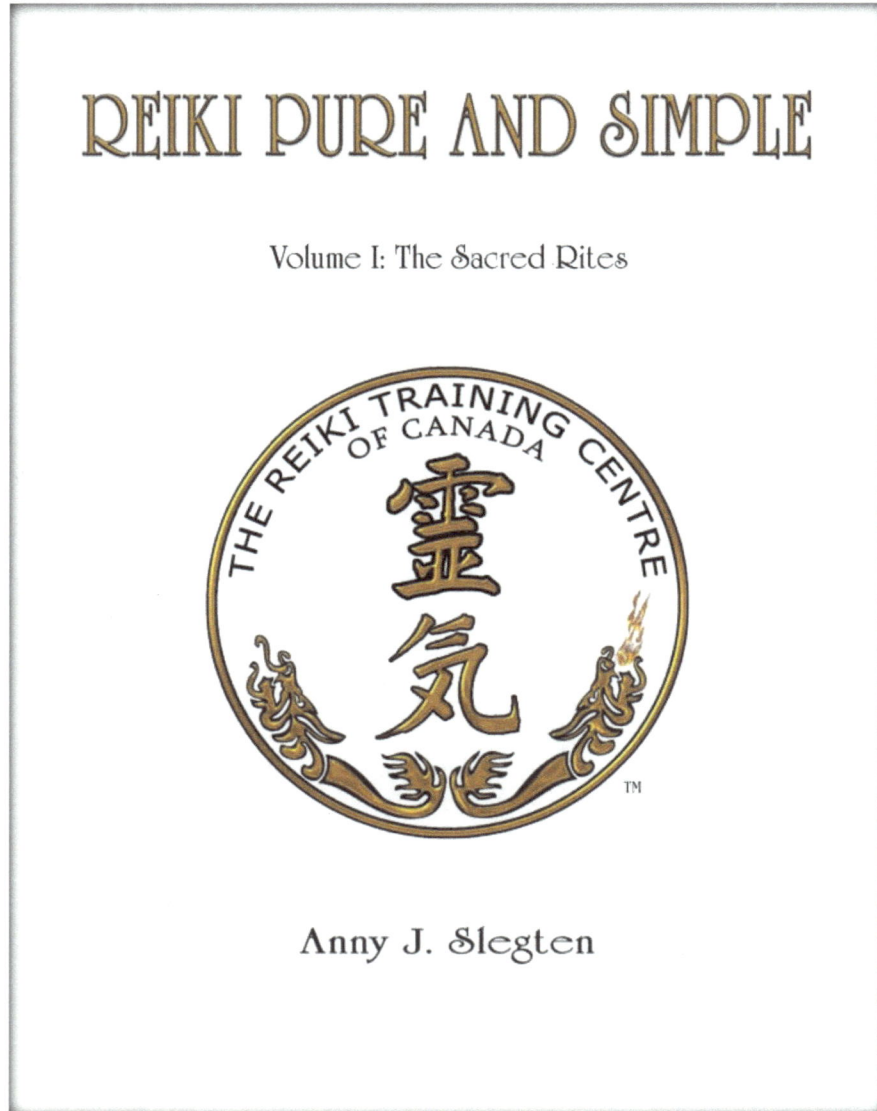

THE REIKI TRAINING CENTRE OF CANADA

靈氣

TM

Anny J. Slegten

Reiki Training Centre of Canada
Class Material
http://www.reiki-canada.com

REIKI PURE AND SIMPLE

Volume II: Reiki Ryoho Hikkei
(The Most Important Methods for Reiki)

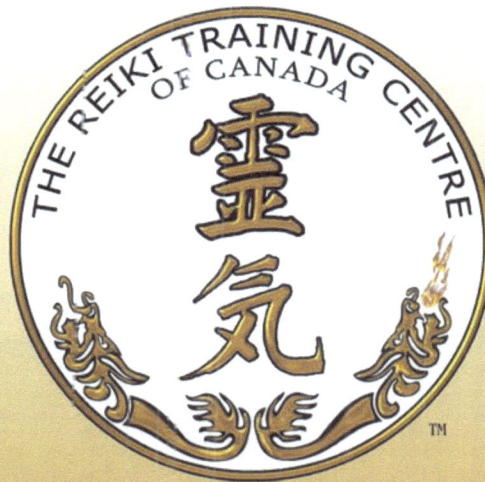

霊気療法必携

Anny J. Slegten

This book is a must read for Reiki Practitioners
regardless of their spiritual lineage
and could be of great benefit to Energy Healers
http://www.reiki-canada.com

REIKI PURE AND SIMPLE

Volume III: The Many Ways of Reiki

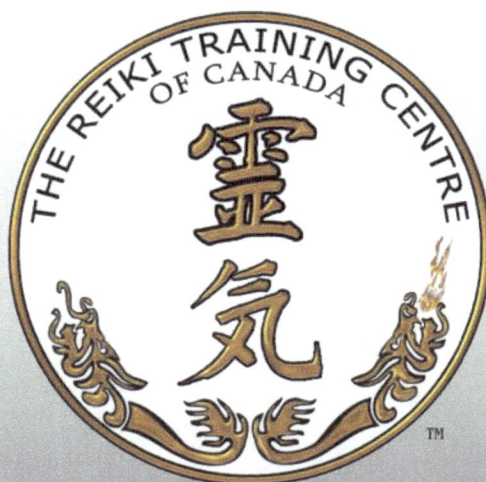

THE REIKI TRAINING CENTRE OF CANADA

霊気

Anny J. Slegten

The Many Ways of Reiki
http://www.reiki-canada.com

REIKI PURE AND SIMPLE

TRADITIONAL JAPANESE REIKI

Volume IV: The Teacher Manual

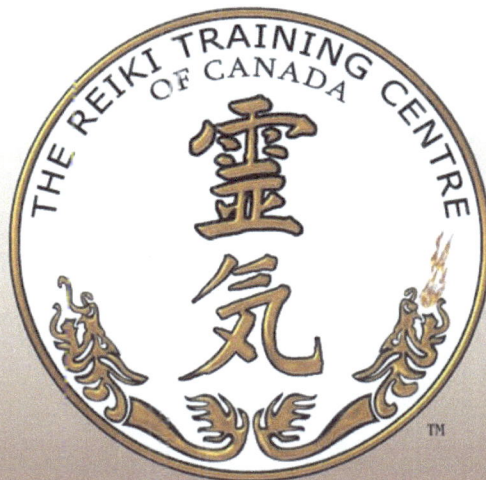

THE REIKI TRAINING CENTRE OF CANADA

靈氣

™

Anny J. Slegten

The Reiki Training Centre of Canada
Teacher's Manual
http://www.reiki-canada.com

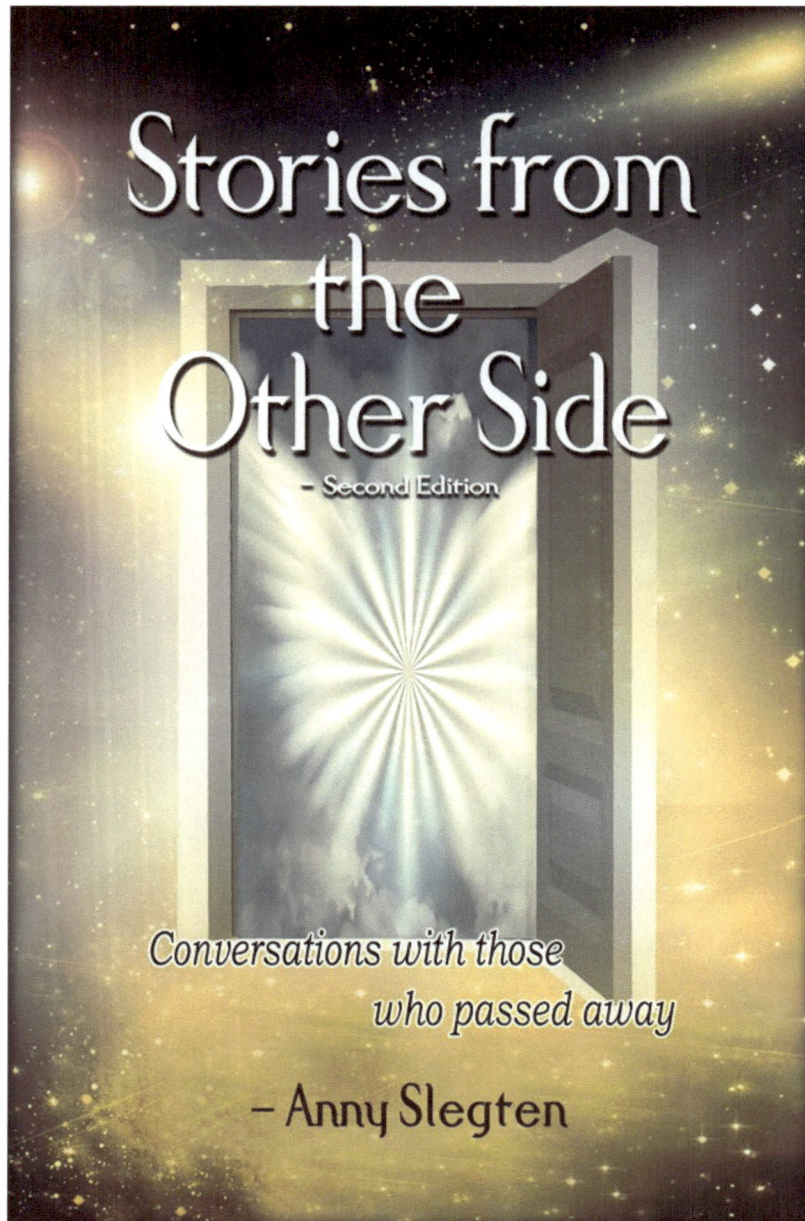

Stories from The Other Side – Second Edition
http://www.connectwithanny.com

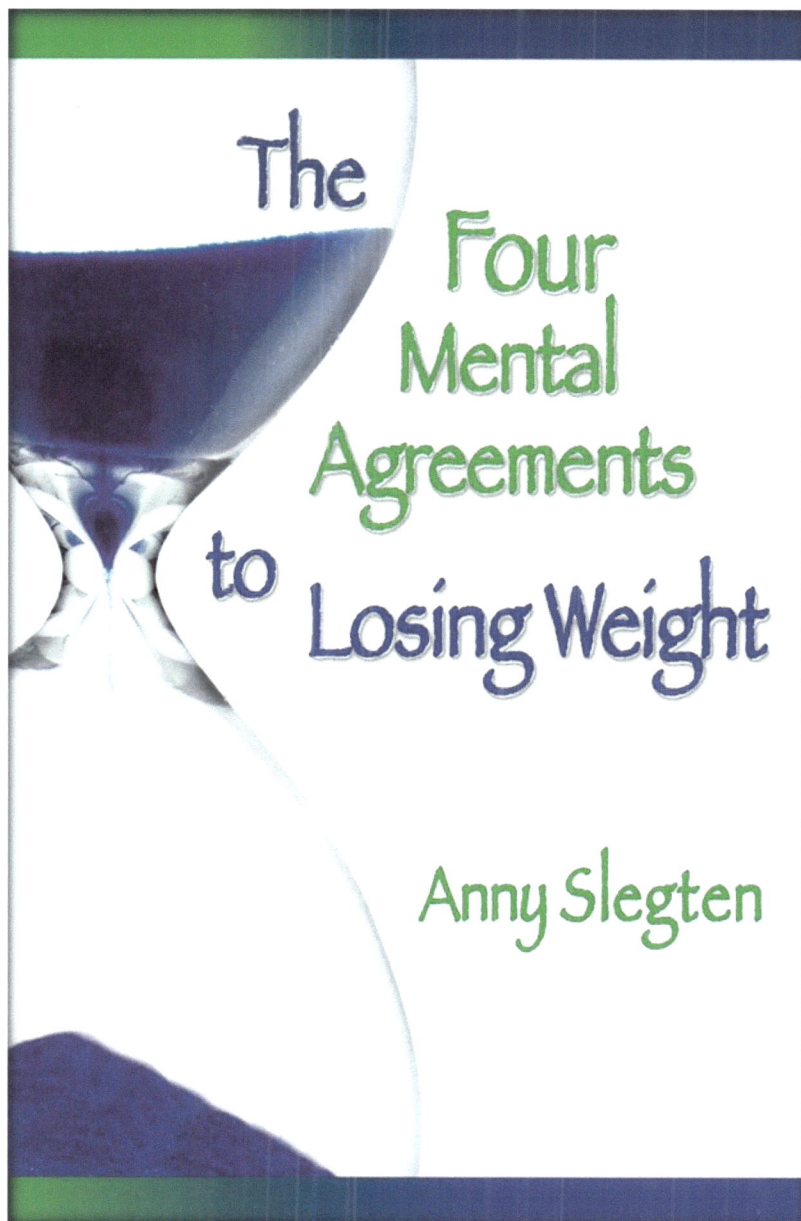

The Four Mental Agreements
To Losing Weight
http://www.connectwithanny.com

www.success-and-more.com

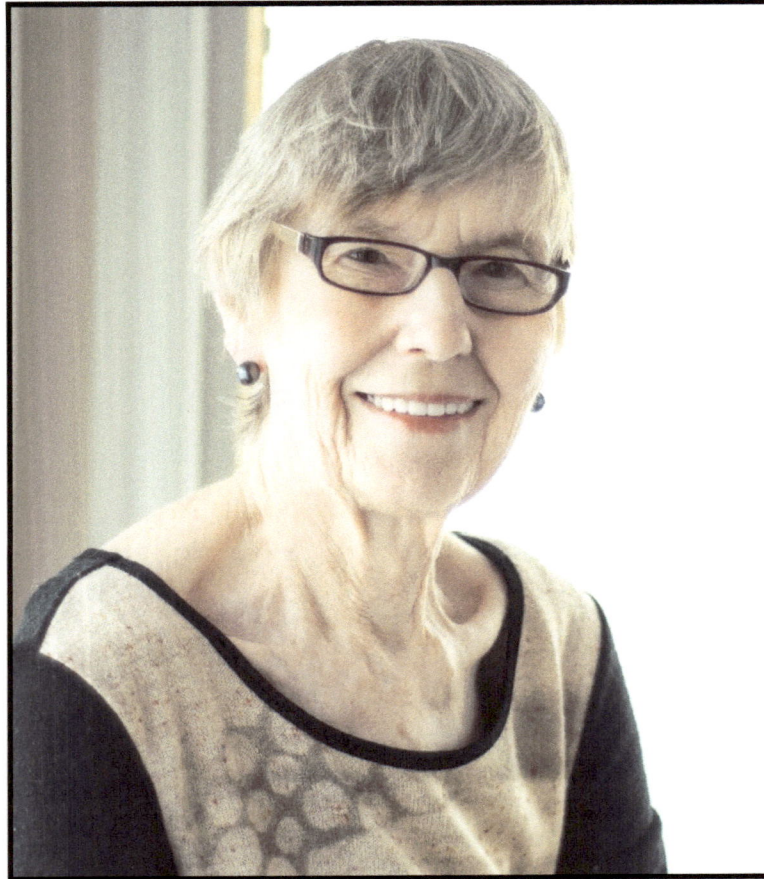

About The Author

As Director of The Hypnotism Training Institute of Alberta and The Reiki Training Centre of Canada, Anny has developed and structured the training and curriculum to the highest standards for both The Hypnotism Training Institute of Alberta and the Reiki Training Centre of Canada.

She offers training to students that come from all over Canada and around the world.

Anny has experienced and lived in many corners of the globe and this has given her a unique understanding of many cultures.

Anny's Belgian parents were from the Flemish part of Belgium and were

    www.success-and-more.com

speaking Flemish (Dutch) at home. Living in Congo, everything was in French.

Although she never spoke Flemish (Dutch), Anny speaks English with a guttural Dutch/German accent. Living in the English-speaking part of Canada for decades, Anny now speaks French with an English accent!

Anny is an Author and holds certifications as:

Master Hypnotist
Clinical Hypnotherapist
Hypno-Baby Birthing Facilitator and Instructor
HypnoBirthing™ Fertility Therapist for Men & Women
Reiki Master/Teacher
Master Remote Viewer

Anny is a world renowned Clinical Hypnotherapist and Hypnologist in full time practice since 1984 as well as a Hypno-Energy worker since 2008.

In 1986 Anny created and developed an unique method using hypnosis for distance services - Virtual Sessions.

Over the years these Virtual Sessions proved to be an effective, useful, and efficient method for investigations and putting closure on both present and past issues - resulting in peace of mind.

To know more about Anny, please visit www.annyslegten.com and make sure to read what she published on her Blog.

Do you wonder what else Anny is publishing?

Visit www.connectwithanny.com

www.ingramcontent.com/pod-product-compliance
Lightning Source LLC
Chambersburg PA
CBHW050814220326
41598CB00006B/202